Daniel Sundfeld Spiga Real

Facial Plastic Surgery

Daniel Sundfeld Spiga Real

Facial Plastic Surgery

The Secrets of Harmonisation

ScienciaScripts

Imprint
Any brand names and product names mentioned in this book are subject to trademark, brand or patent protection and are trademarks or registered trademarks of their respective holders. The use of brand names, product names, common names, trade names, product descriptions etc. even without a particular marking in this work is in no way to be construed to mean that such names may be regarded as unrestricted in respect of trademark and brand protection legislation and could thus be used by anyone.

Cover image: www.ingimage.com

This book is a translation from the original published under ISBN 978-613-9-64722-4.

Publisher:
Sciencia Scripts
is a trademark of
Dodo Books Indian Ocean Ltd. and OmniScriptum S.R.L publishing group

120 High Road, East Finchley, London, N2 9ED, United Kingdom
Str. Armeneasca 28/1, office 1, Chisinau MD-2012, Republic of Moldova, Europe
Printed at: see last page
ISBN: 978-620-7-78125-6

Foreword

Plastic Surgery is a medical speciality that is close to the most beautiful and solemn arts. Interspersed with painting and, above all, sculpture, this speciality brings synesthesia to sounds, flavours and images, transforming them into surgical procedures that seek the physical and psychological harmonisation of patients.

The archetype of Plastic Surgery lies in the desire of the first surgeons to re-establish proportions and harmony in patients with mutilations caused by trauma and/or disease, with a view to the aesthetics and functionality of the reconstructed parts.

Nowadays, there are huge obstacles in the way of dividing plastic surgery into aesthetic and restorative, which are even taken to court as legal claims in an attempt to hold professionals accountable for a medicine that is an end and not a means.

This discussion is unfounded, as plastic surgery arose from the need for repair, and to this day continues to have the same objectives, since even in a procedure considered to be aesthetic, the desired outcome is the repair of a diagnosis made with the correct proposition of treatment in the search for harmonisation of proportions and functionality.

From this perspective, this work aims to provide a review of the literature as well as the author's contributions to the advancement and development of Plastic Surgery, especially in the aspects that circumscribe facial surgeries, since the face is the part of our body that has the most functions, serving as a mirror of our emotions, feelings and showing our life story with the forging of the years in our expression marks and positioning of facial structures in their various compartments.Without the slightest pretence of exhausting the myriad of knowledge about facial plastic surgery, I hope that you, noble reader, will enjoy this brief review quoting great surgeons and their techniques, dealing with otoplasty and surgery to treat disorders of the upper third of the face, specifically ptosis of the tail of the eyebrow and orbito-palpebral rejuvenation.

A good journey into the marvellous world of Facial Plastic Surgery!

Yours faithfully Dr Daniel Sundfeld Spiga Real

Thank you

> "A dream that is dreamt alone is just a dream that is dreamt alone, but a dream that is dreamt together is reality" (Prelude - Raul Seixas).
>
> "A dream you dream alone is only a dream. A dream you dream together is reality" (John Lennon).

The great achievements forged in human history have always been achieved through the co-operation of individuals who believed in an ideal and came together to realise it.

Therefore, as an honour, I would like to express my sincere thanks to the patients who took part in the studies, to the residents and colleagues who helped in all the processes of structuring and carrying out the projects. I am grateful to my glorious Paulista School of Medicine, which was responsible for all my training and opportunities to develop in my profession. I would also like to highlight the Plastic Surgery Discipline in the form of Prof³ Dr³ Lydia Masako Ferreira, the great promoter of the scientific productions discussed here.

My special thanks go to my family, especially my wife Mônica, who has inspired and encouraged me throughout my life and achievements!

Thank you very much!

Summary

CHAPTER 1

Otoplasty: the art of harmonising the auricle

Sundfeld-Reis point*

Dr Daniel Sundfeld Spiga Real

***Article Published in the Brazilian Journal of Plastic Surgery**
- Rev. Bras. Cir. Plást. 2013;28(3):493-498

Historically, enduring the centuries, the face has been portrayed as one of the main means of communication, characterising the backdrop for expressions of feelings and emotions. This can be seen in famous works such as Leonardo da Vinci's "La Gioconda" from 1503-1506, part of the Italian Renaissance movement, and Edvard Munch's "The Scream (Skrik)" from 1893, part of Expressionism.

As part of its composition and largely responsible for its harmony, the external ear is a source of great stigma in society. Prominent ears are the most common congenital deformity of the external ear, affecting approximately 5% of the general population[1] . Transmitted in an autosomal dominant manner, despite the benign physiological consequences, many studies have shown the psychological suffering, emotional trauma and changes in behaviour that this deformity can cause, especially in children .[2]

In the literature there is a wide range of techniques for the correction of prominent ears that can be grouped into techniques: with incision and suture[3] , suture only[4] , techniques with cartilage removal[5-7] , and others that combine some of the aforementioned[8] .

The current state of the art suggests that there is no one ideal method for correcting prominent ears and that there is still room for new developments.

In otoplasty, good surgical results require knowledge of the embryology and anatomy of the external ear.
The pinna develops from six mesenchymal proliferations around the fifth week of gestation known as promontories of His. These are located in the dorsal region of the first and second branchial arches. Later, the promontories fuse around the dorsal region of the first pharyngeal cleft, forming the auricular pavilion.

Each promontory contributes to the formation of a specific outer ear structure. As foetal development progresses, the external ear migrates from the cervical region to the side of the skull[9] .

The sensory and motor innervation of the external ear is represented by the following nerves: vagus nerve (X) - auricular branch; great auricular nerve with its anterior and posterior branches (C2/C3); mandibular nerve (V); auriculotemporal nerve; external acoustic meatus nerve; facial nerve (VII) - auricular branch, and posterior auricular nerve responsible for innervating the muscles of the external ear[10] . The external ear is a complex structure made up mainly of skin and cartilage, formed by five main elements: concha, helix, antelix, tragus and lobe. Other portions, of lesser importance, are: antitragus, intertragal sulcus and Darwin's tubercle (Fig.1).

The division of the ear can be understood embryologically through the gill arches. The second branchial arch is the main contributor to the formation of the ear, contributing to the formation of the helix, scapus, antelix, concha, antitragus and lobe, while the first branchial arch only contributes to the formation of the tragus and crus helix.

The innervation of the external ear, as shown above, follows the distribution of the branchial arches and consists of the anterior and posterior branches of the greater auricular nerve, which innervates the structures originating from the first branchial arch (tragus and crus helix), and the auriculotemporal nerve, which innervates the structures originating from the second branchial arch (helix, scaphoid, antelix, concha, antitragus, external acoustic meatus, and lobe). The external acoustic meatus also receives innervation from branches of the vagus and glossopharyngeal nerves[11] .

Irrigation is via the posterior auricular and occipital branches of the external carotid artery and the anterior auricular branch of the superficial temporal artery. The auricular pavilion has several ligaments and muscles, including the greater helix muscle, the lesser helix muscle, the tragus muscle and the antitragus muscle. Its posterior surface includes the superior auricular ligament, the oblique ear muscle, the transverse ear muscle and the posterior auricular ligament[10] .

The ideal positioning of the external ear in relation to the other components of the face contributes to harmony and an ideal aesthetic appearance. From an anteroposterior perspective, the desired auriculocephalic angle should be between 15 and 30 degrees, with 25 to 30 degrees considered ideal. The distance from the edge of the helix to the mastoid should be between 15 and 20mm. The vertical orientation of the pinna should be strictly parallel to the nasal dorsum. A horizontal line extending from the inferior orbital margin should be at the same level as the upper edge of the tragus[12] .

Other parameters used to characterise prominent ears are the measurements from the lateral edge of the helix to the temporal region and mastoid, on a perpendicular line, with values ranging from: upper pole: 10 to 12 mm; middle portion: 15 to 25 mm; and lower pole from 20 to 22 mm, with these measurements varying greatly according to the physical type, racial group and age of the patient[13] .

The main causes of prominent ears include: (1) excess or hypertrophy of the concha (upper pole, lower pole or both); (2) inadequate formation of the antelix projection (antelix base, upper crus, lower crus or all); (3) a scapho-conchal angle greater than 90 degrees; and (4) a combination of concha hypertrophy and incomplete development of the antelix. Other causes can include cranial abnormalities (which can influence the assessment of the base on which the ear rests), lobe protrusion and anterolateral displacement of the helix tail[14] .

It is clear from the above that, despite the many techniques in the literature, there is no consensus on which is the ideal method for performing otoplasty, with many techniques receiving numerous variations and withstanding the test of time. Consequently, the Sundfeld-Reis technique using the helix branch stitch aims to add a new surgical technique for better composition and harmony in otoplasty, as it is a simple technique with known complications.

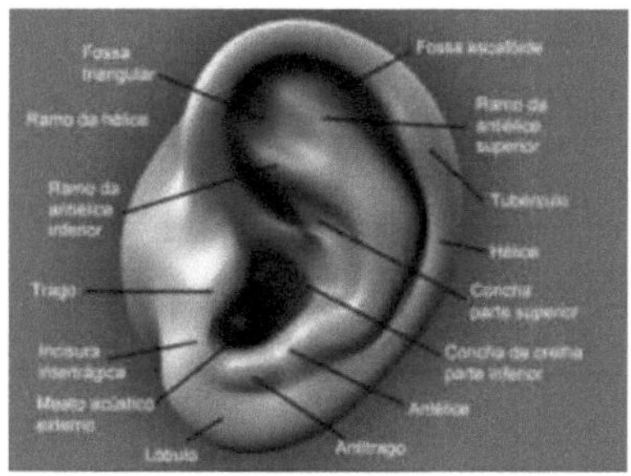

(Figure.1)

Technique Description

Firstly, markings are made on the anterior and posterior surfaces of the outer ear, demarcating the locations of the Sundfeld-Reis points.

Positioned in the supine position, after antisepsis with aqueous chlorhexidine, they are submitted to local anaesthesia with anaesthetic solution (Lidocaine 2% - 40 ml without vasoconstrictor, isotonic saline solution 60 ml, adrenaline 0.5 ml, resulting in a 1:200,000 solution). Infiltration of anaesthetic in the subcutaneous plane along the posterior and anterior portions and in the anterior portion of the external acoustic meatus for a total anaesthetic block. Wait approximately 10 minutes for vasoconstriction to reach its peak due to the local effect of the injected adrenaline. No sedation of any kind is used.

Sterile drapes, positioned on the head, allowing lateral rotation with exposure of the ears for comparison and symmetry in the repair results. For greater safety and to prevent infectious complications, due to the large area of detachment and manipulation, first generation cephalosporins are used as antibiotic therapy for seven days post-operatively.

After excising the spindle of skin from the posterior portion of the ear, dissected up to the plane of the posterior perichondrium, dissection is carried out up to the edge of the helix along the entire length of the pinna. This is followed by dissection of the mastoid and then strict haemostasis.

Next, the technique proposed by this author of making a stitch with black Mononylon 3.0 on the portion of the Helix Branch, in the region known as the crus helix, between the upper (Cymba of concha) and lower (Cavum of concha) shells, as shown in figure 2, here called the Sundfeld-Reis stitch.

After this point, the effects are observed (Figure 3). If the upper pole of the outer ear is already in a harmonic position and its vertical axis is parallel to the dorsum of the nose, the Mustardé stitch is continued with colourless Mononylon 4.0 to make the antelix and Furnas with black Mononylon 3.0.

The above-mentioned procedures are repeated in the contralateral ear and, at the end, they are compared in terms of symmetry. The posterior incisions are sutured with black Mononylon 5.0 in a continuous suture, after a further review of haemostasis.

Contensive bandaging is performed, with the outer ear moulded with sterile cotton wool. This is removed on the first post-operative day and replaced with an elasticated otoplasty bandage.

Patients are followed up at regular intervals. At every visit, patients are photographed for later comparison.

At these returns, the occurrence of complications such as infection, haematomas, tissue necrosis, pressure injuries, paresthesia, suture dehiscence, recurrence of the prominence and thread extrusion are assessed.

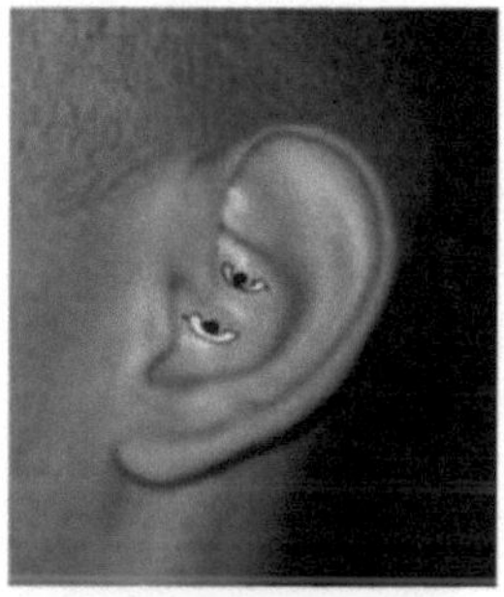

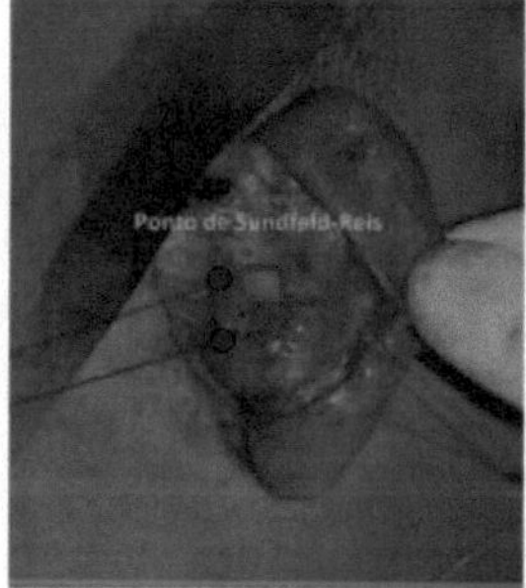

(Figura 2).

(Making the Sundfeld-Reis stitch).

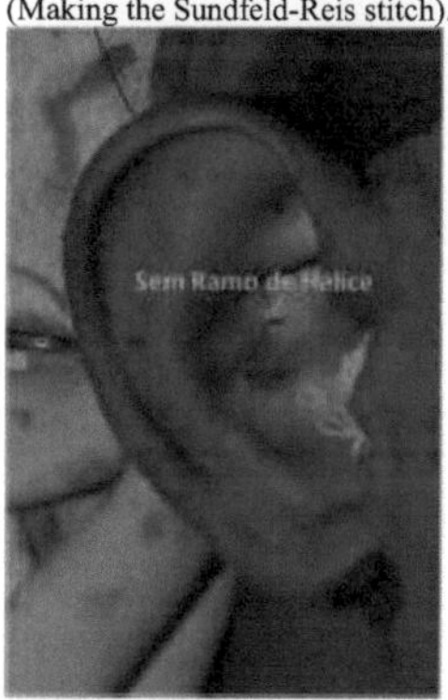

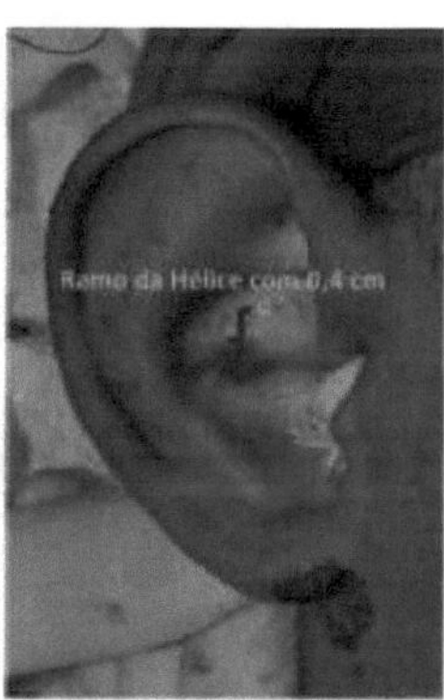

(External ear without the tension of the Sundfeld-Reis point). (External ear showing the effect of the Sundfeld-Reis point).

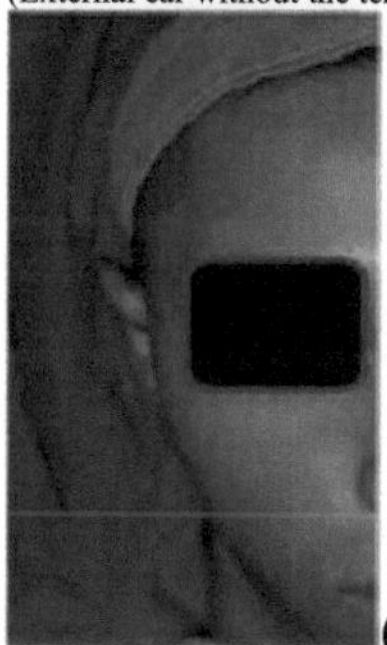

(Figure 3).

(Aspect of the external ear after Sundfeld-Reis stitches).

In the first six months of follow-up, no recurrence, dehiscence, infection, haematoma, cartilage and/or tissue necrosis were observed (Figure 4). Complaints of a slight sensation of paresthesia in the auricular region were noted in 33% of patients after three months.

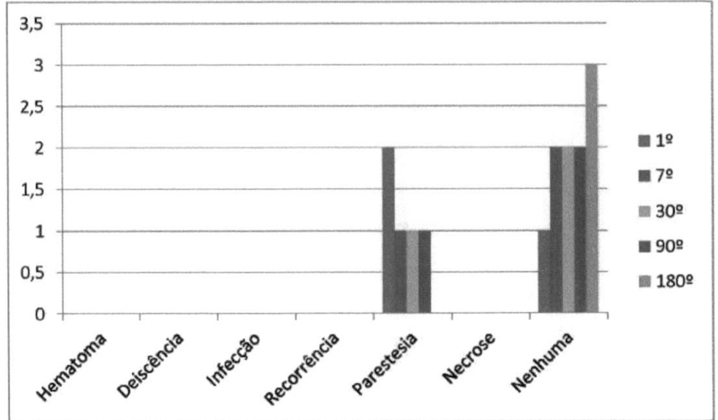

Complications versus observation time

(Figure 4)

Literature Review

Forged by time, the different otoplasty techniques have transcended the centuries and are becoming more and more topical. In 1845, Dieffenbach described the first case of otoplasty performed on a patient with post-traumatic sequelae. He performed post-auricular skin resection and conchomastoid fixation as a form of treatment[15] .

Ely described his technique for elective otoplasties in 1881, in which he performed excision of the post-auricular skin, conchomastoid fixation and excision of a strip of conchal cartilage. The procedure was carried out in two surgical procedures[16] .

Analysing the literature reviews carried out by Keen, Cocheril, and

Gersuny; Luckett highlighted the importance of making and restoring the shape of the antelix in the otoplasty procedure[17] . Luckett also introduced the revolutionary concept of manipulating the auricular cartilage to achieve a natural shape. In creating the antelix, he used a posterior access and resected the cartilage with subsequent union of the edges. In 1952, Becker introduced a concept for obtaining a smoother shape for the antelix, using incisions in the cartilage associated with sutures[18] .

Mustardé's 1963 approach to creating a new antelix was based on permanent sutures via a posterior access and the stitches encompassed up to the anterior perichondrium, without transfixing the skin[4] .

Stenstrom (1963) developed his technique using anterior scraping to achieve a smoother contour of the antelix[5] . With regard to concha deformities, there are various forms of correction, including excision, scraping and cartilage fixation. Suture techniques were first described by Owens and Delgado(1955)[19] .

Furnas, in 1968, modified Owens and Delgado's technique by suturing with a non-absorbable thread positioned in the conchal cartilage, transfixed up to the anterior perichondrium and sutured to the mastoid fascia[20] .

The Furnas technique had achieved great popularity due to its simplicity and easy reproduction, but like many other techniques, it was modified by Spira et al in 1969[21] .

The Sundfeld-Reis technique offers a simple solution for correcting the upper auricular pole and the auricular axis, with complication rates comparable to those in the literature. It offers harmonious aesthetic results and a low or no recurrence rate.

Furthermore, the Sundfeld-Reis approach is not similar to any other technique described in the literature. It is simple and easily reproducible, with satisfactory long-term results and improved facial harmony.

The technique described as Sundfeld-Reis, with the point made in the Helix Branch, represents a simple and reproducible way of correcting the upper pole and the auricular axis, making it parallel to the nasal dorsum, without the need for the point made in the triangular fossa and temporal fascia, as envisaged by Adamson et al[22] for correction of the upper pole, as well as not encouraging complication rates.

The spectacular world of otoplasty represents a great challenge for the most skilful surgeons. Numerous techniques have been and are described in the literature, always seeking the best way to achieve the best facial harmony, but since the pinna is a structure with many peculiarities, we have not yet managed to develop the ideal technique for all cases of prominent ears.

Each case must be assessed individually and it is up to the plastic surgeon, within his arsenal of knowledge, to indicate the best form of treatment, using the best technique for the specific case. As such, there is a lot of progress to be made in surgery to correct prominent ears, and this author proposes that further studies be carried out, and who knows, maybe one day the ideal procedure for facial and pinna harmonisation will be achieved.

Example of a case operated with the Sundfeld-Reis Point

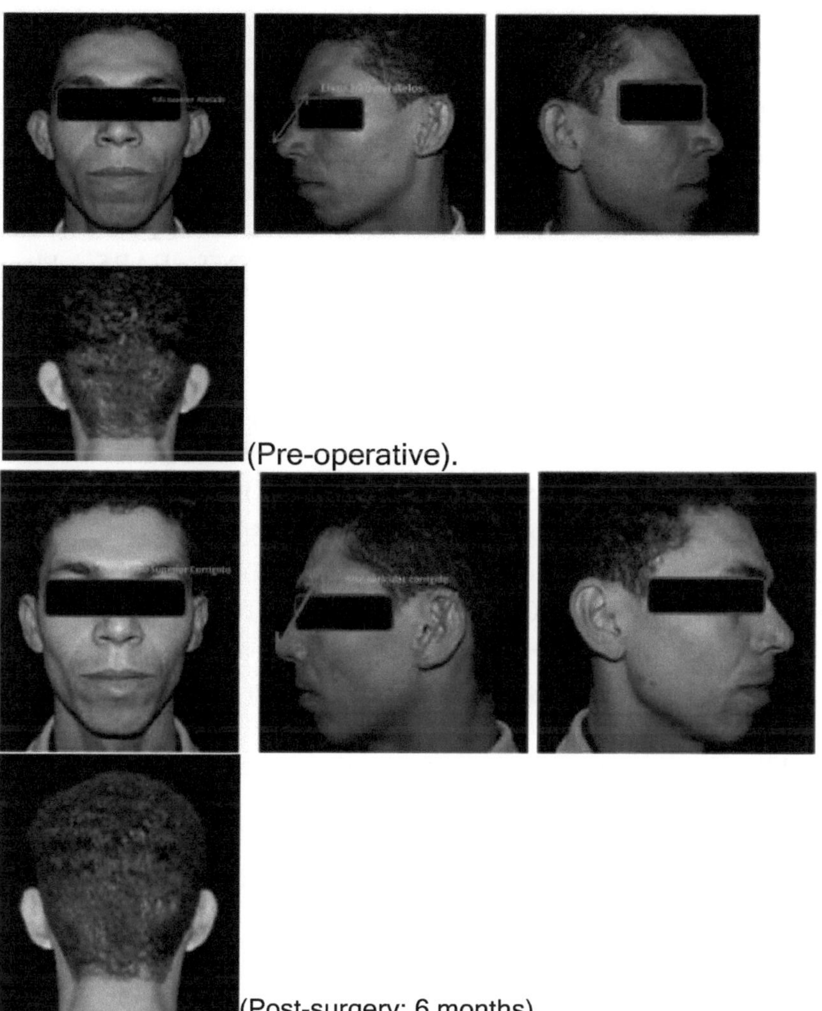

(Pre-operative).

(Post-surgery: 6 months).

Bibliography

1- Janis JE, Rohrich RJ, Gutowski KA. Otoplasty. Plast Reconstr Surg. 2005 Apr;115(4):60e 72e.

2- - Macgregor FC. Ear deformities: social and psychological implications. Clin Plast Surg. 1978 Jul;5(3):347-50.

3- CONVERSE JM, NIGRO A, WILSON FA, JOHNSON N. A technique for surgical
correction of lop ears. Plast Reconstr Surg (1946). 1955 May;15(5):411-8.

4- MUSTARDE JC. The correction of prominent ears using simple mattress sutures.Br J Plast Surg. 1963 Apr;16:170-8.

5- STENSTROEM SJ. A "NATURAL" TECHNIQUE FOR CORRECTION OF CONGENITALLY PROMINENT EARS. Plast Reconstr Surg. 1963 Nov;32:509-18.

6- JU DM, LI C, CRIKELAIR GF. THE SURGICAL CORRECTION OF PROTRUDING EARS. Plast Reconstr Surg. 1963 Sep;32:283-93.

7- CHONGCHET V. A METHOD OF ANTIHELIX RECONSTRUCTION. Br J Plast Surg. 1963 Jul;16:268-72.

8- Schlegel-Wagner C, Pabst G, Muller W, Linder T. Otoplasty using a modified anterior scoring technique: standardised measurements of long-term results. Arch Facial Plast Surg. 2010 May-Jun;12(3):143-8.

9- Sadler TW. Ear (chapter 17), in ***Lengman's*** Med/ca/ ***Embiyology*** (ed. 6). Baltimore, MD, Williams & Wilkins, 1990.

10- Sobotta, Atlas of Human Anatomy, Vol.1,382-383, 21[a] Guanabara Koogan Edition, 2000.

11- Tolleth H. Artistic anatomy, dimensions, and proportions of the external ear.Clin Plast Surg. 1978 Jul;5(3):337-45.

12- Spira M. Otoplasty: what I do now--a 30-year perspective. Plast Reconstr Surg.1999 Sep;104(3):834-40; discussion 841.

13- Stucker FJ, Vora NM, Lian TS. Otoplasty: an analysis of technique over a 33-year period. Laryngoscope. 2003 Jun;113(6):952-6.

14- Webster GV. The tail of the helix as a key to otoplasty. Plast Reconstr Surg.1969 Nov;44(5):455-61.

15- Dieffenbach, JE. Die operative chirurgie. Leipzig: F. A. Brockhause, 1845.

16- Ely, ET. An operation for prominet auricles. Arch. Otolaryngol.1881; 10:97, (reprinted in Plast. Reconst. Surg.1968; 42: 582).

17- Rogers BO. The classic reprint. A New Operation for Prominent Ears Based on the Anatomy of the Deformity by William H. Luckett, M.D. (reprinted from Surg.Gynec. & Obst., 10: 635-7, 1910). Plast Reconstr Surg. 1969 Jan;43(1):83-6.

18- BECKER OJ. Correction of the protruding deformed ear. Br J Plast Surg. 1952 Oct;5(3):187-96.

19- OWENS N, DELGADO DD. THE MANAGEMENT OF OUTSTANDING EARS. South Med J. 1965 Jan;58:32-3.

20- Furnas DW. Correction of prominent ears by conchamastoid sutures. Plast Reconstr Surg. 1968 Sep;42(3):189-93.

21- Spira M, McCrea R, Gerow FJ, Hardy SB. Correction of the principal deformities causing protruding ears. Plast Reconstr Surg. 1969 Aug;44(2):150-4.

22- Adamson PA, McGraw BL, Tropper GJ. Otoplasty: critical review of clinical results. Laryngoscope. 1991 Aug;101(8):883-8.

CHAPTER 2

Facial ageing

Clinical Classification of the Degree of Ptosis of the Superciliary Tail

Dr Daniel Sundfeld Spiga Real

***Article Published in the Brazilian Journal of Plastic Surgery**
- Rev. Bras. Cir. Plast. 2016;31(3):354-361

Throughout the centuries, beauty has been one of the main motifs and challenges for the geniuses of the arts. With regard to the classical ideal of human beauty, sages and artists have been searching for a way to represent it since the dawn of time. An example of this is the work of Marco Vitruvio Polião, the famous Roman architect who described the perfection of the human body with measurements and proportions, denoting them in relation to the so-called "golden ratio"[1] .

This work, which only expressed the proportions of the human body in numbers, was portrayed by a brilliant Renaissance artist who immortalised the "Human Being" in his works. Leonardo Da Vinci, in "Vitruvian Man", materialises numbers on the human body, demonstrating the proportions of beauty. Another important manifestation of Da Vinci's genius is framed in "La Gioconda", where classical beauty is demonstrated in the proportions of the face and, above all, in the expressions of the gaze.

As an archetype, human beauty is represented mainly in the face, with all its nuances and expressions of feelings, as well as the appearance of the body's ageing stages. This demonstrates the great importance of facial expressions and the proportions of their constituents in men's social relationships and health.

Scientifically, ageing is portrayed by the repositioning of facial structures, both in their soft tissue components and in their bone framework, as defined in studies carried out by Shaw RB et al (2011)[2] and Matros E et al (2009)[3] , studies carried out using measurements in photographic records and CT scans with 3D reconstruction, which showed bone and volume changes in the face and the repositioning of the supercilium in its central medial and medial portions, respectively.

In this context, the eyebrows, especially their tail, represent, through their movements and placement, the sector with the greatest capacity to portray an individual's feelings as well as their ageing, as well characterised by writer and artist Gordon C. Aymar: "the eyes are the place where the most complete, reliable and pertinent information about the subject is seen. And the eyebrow can register, almost single-handedly, wonder, pity, fear, pain, cynicism, concentration, nostalgia, displeasure and hope, in infinite variations and combinations"[4] .

From this preamble, the study of the eyebrow has become a major challenge for plastic surgery, since one of the main aims of this medical speciality is to define classic beauty by adjusting the proportions of facial areas and repositioning structures, aiming for a youthful and empathetic expression. After reviewing the literature in the main databases, many studies permeate the evaluation and treatment of the tail of the eyebrow[5,6,7,8,9,10,11,12] , but there are no studies whose motto is the classification of the ptosis of this anatomical structure and, based on this, suggest the treatment of the region to readjust the beauty proportions of the face.

Classification Description

To carry out the classification, groups of patients were recruited from different age groups. Their measurements were taken by different observers and characterised after statistical studies, as outlined below.

The measurement was carried out directly and objectively on the patients during the facial physical examination, with the patients in an orthostatic position with a neutral gaze fixed on the horizon and with the facial muscles relaxed. Three measurements were taken on each side by different examiners, totalling nine measurements on each side, without each person knowing the value of the other's measurement.

A digital caliper (precision 0.01mm; OTMT Machines, NY, USA) was used to measure the end point of the supercilium (FS) to the Frankfurt plane (PF) (Figure 1), delimiting a line (X) that connects these points and makes a 90° angle with the Frankfurt plane (Figures 2a and 2b).

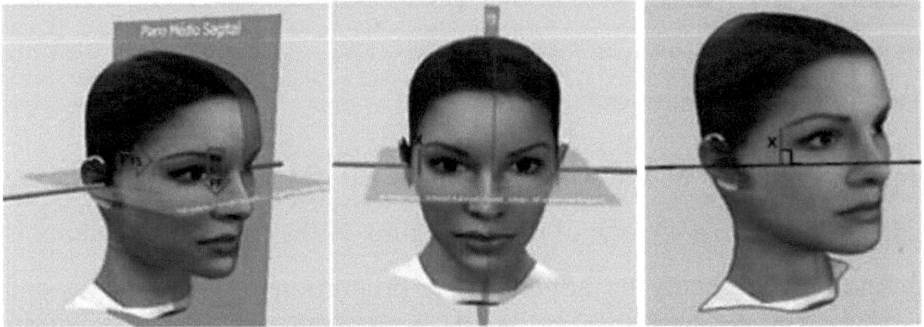

(Figure 1) Demonstration of the End Point of the Superciliary Tail (FS) and the Frankfurt Plane (PF).
(Figure 2a) Demonstration of the Line (X) perpendicular to the Frankfurt Plane - frontal view.
(Line (X) perpendicular to the Frankfurt Plane - lateral view.

The Frankfurt Plane is defined as the plane established by the lowest point of the orbital margin to the highest point of the external auditory canal[13], which is an important anatomical reference and easy for plastic surgeons to define in their facial examinations.

The resulting quantitative data from the measurements was subjected to statistical analyses using Student's t-test in each group and inter-group comparisons were made using the non-parametric Wilcoxon test. A table classifying the degrees of ptosis was drawn up with the data and suggestions for surgical intervention according to clinical manifestation.

The clinical classification of ptosis of the tail of the eyebrow is a great help to plastic surgeons, as it emphasises the importance of a correct diagnosis and an appropriate surgical proposal, avoiding upper blepharoplasty surgeries without the proper indication and with unsatisfactory results due to incorrect or deficient diagnoses.

After analysing all this data, Table 5 was created, which corresponds to the classification proposed in this study. It should be noted that all the data was analysed for its intra-group and inter-group differences, allowing these conclusions to be ratified. The statistical statements below Table 1 show the validity of the data presented.

DISTANCE (CM).	DEGREE OF PTOSIS.	INDICATION FOR SURGERY.
≥1,8	NORMAL	NO
17-1,5	I	NO
1,4-1,2	II	YES
1,1 -0,9	III	YES
≤0,8	IV	YES

Table 1. Classification of Ptosis of the Superciliary Tail vs Surgical Indication.

Literature Review

Forged over centuries, the need for classifications has permeated the evolution of humanity. Since the beginning, man has used classifications for his social organisation. The oldest known system of classification was carried out by Aristotle, who dichotomised living beings into animals and plants[14] .

In today's world, this need is becoming more and more apparent, as the amount of new knowledge that emerges on a daily basis would not be used if it were not classified and organised. Looking through the literature, there are several articles that propose ways of measuring the positioning of the supercilia[5,6,12] and ways of evaluating them through standardised image captures[15] , but none of them present an objective way of doing this, with defined anatomical points, nor do they present a clinical classification that provides the plastic surgeon with an assessment of their patient when determining an intervention.

Taking as its archetype the need to carry out a simple measurement based on points with little individual variation (bone structures), the present study outlined the Frankfurt Plane as the basic reference for measurement, as this plane is easy to characterise without the need for sophisticated instruments. This characteristic makes the measurement of the end of the tail of the eyebrow to the Frankfurt plane in a perpendicular line an ideal tool that is easy to apply for assessing this region in the plastic surgeon's physical examination.

The proposal presented in this study to use measurements subdivided by age group, with group 1 (n=30, 18 - 30 years) used as normal values and the other groups 2 (n=30, 30 - 60 years) and 3 (n=30, 61 - 100 years) as varying degrees of ptosis, denotes the data found in the literature which shows that the characteristics of the skin are maintained up to the age of 30, with sequential changes of greater loss of collagen and destructuring of the dermal matrix up to the age of 60 and, after that, a faster evolution[16,17] , resulting in greater ptosis. Hwang.K (2013)[16] showed in his study of the Korean population that the thickness of the epidermis and dermis of the eyelid and brow region thinned with advancing age, with average values of 884pm at the age of 30 and 818pm at the age of 61 or over. This justifies and ratifies the values found for ptosis of the tail of the eyebrow, since after the age of 30 the values were lower and after the age of 61 these differences were more discrepant in relation to the younger groups.

When the measurement data was analysed, it was found that the measurements of group 1, considered normal, with a mean age of 26.7 years, ranged from 1.6 cm to 2.7 cm, with a mean of 2.14 cm, median of 2.2 cm and mode of 2.2 cm in relation to measurements of ptosis of the tail of the eyebrow. In group 2, the mean age was 44.2 years and the variation ranged from 1.2 cm to 2.5 cm, with a mean of 1.9 cm, median of 1.98 cm and mode of 2.1 cm, showing a tendency towards ptosis due to age-related changes. Corresponding to group 3, the data analysis described the histological findings of changes in the skin, showing a mean age of 72.6 years and a variation of 0.5 cm to 1.93 cm, with a mean of 1.27 cm, median of 1.4 cm and mode of 1.2 cm in relation to measurements of ptosis of the tail of the eyebrow.

There are no studies in the literature that measure and analyse the above methods, which does not allow for correspondence with other publications. Packiriswamy.V et. al (2013)[6] , carried out a study with a population of 400 individuals aged between 18 and 26 from Malaysia or South India to try to determine whether there were differences between the positions of the superciliums in these populations. The method used was through measurements taken on photographs and the fall of the tail of the eyebrow was measured using an oblique line between the lateral ocular corner and the end of the eyebrow. As a result, they found that there was no difference between the populations, with the average male measurements being 16.25 ± 2.39 mm in the Malays and 16.09 ± 2.29 mm in the South Indians. In the female population, they found slightly higher values of 17.15 ± 2.08 mm in the Malasians and 17.58 ± 2.5 mm in the South Indians. This study was limited by the fact that its method used photographs and computer measurements with no fixed anatomical landmarks, and the measurements were taken in just one dimension. Furthermore, the measurements taken to try to demonstrate ptosis of the tail of the eyebrow were based on two mobile points that change with age - the tail and the lateral corner of the orbital fissure - which leads to bias in this measurement.

Matai.O et. Al(2007)[12] described an angular measurement of ptosis of the tail of the eyebrow, using 261 patients, 125 children aged 4 to 6 and 136 adults over 50, subdivided into groups aged 50-60, 61-70 and over 70. All patients were filmed for 3 minutes in a frontal position and the measurements were made using computer programmes. The authors did not describe the values, only that they found a difference between the children and the adult group. This study shows very different age groups, with children still in the growth phase and without formed craniofacial structures. The method of frontal filming and then computer measurements does not make it possible to really measure the end of the tail of the eyebrow, since the face is a three-dimensional structure. The inclusion factors for this study were also not well delineated with very heterogeneous groups, resulting in sample and comparison biases. For these reasons, there was a need to create another measurement method that would make it possible to suggest a treatment based on this classification.

In the study in question, with the above data, statistical calculations were made, with the standard deviation equated at 0.2 points. As such, the values presented were £1.8 cm; 1.7 - 1.5 cm; 1.4 - 1.2 cm; 1.1 - 0.9 cm and < 0.8 cm (Table 5) at intervals of this standard deviation. It should be emphasised that the aim of this study was to present a clinical classification that could be carried out in consultation and that would help professionals to outline their conduct and seek the best positioning of the tail of the eyebrow after surgery.

Jones. BM et al (2013)[7] presented in their study the follow-up of patients undergoing video-assisted frontoplasty over a 5-year period. To do this, they used computer measurements of photos taken of their patients preoperatively and postoperatively, using the pupil as a reference point when looking neutrally and some points marked on the eyebrow, with no fixed reference point for reliable measurement. These characteristics make this study difficult to reproduce and use in the practice of plastic surgeons, as well as not presenting the measurements for a population, but for each individual patient pre- and post-operatively.

This study assigned a degree of ptosis to each interval, ranging from grade I to grade IV, in order to refine the surgeon's perception in his assessment. Each grade was correlated with a numerical interval in which: >1.8 cm represents normality; 1.7-1.5 cm represents grade I ptosis; 1.4 - 1.2 cm represents grade II ptosis; 1.1 - 0.9 cm represents grade III ptosis and < 0.8 cm represents grade IV ptosis. Surgical indication was given for grades II,

III and IV.

Thus, by defining the degree of ptosis of the tail of the eyebrow, it is possible to decide whether or not to proceed with surgery, always matching the objective measurement data with the patient's clinical complaints for the best course of action.

These characteristics and objectives have not been matched by any other publication to date, emphasising the uniqueness of the study with the creation of an unprecedented classification based on objective measurements and well-defined anatomical parameters that are easy to delimit, with minor changes between age groups and ethnicities.

The current study is based on the Brazilian population, which is highly miscegenated and therefore has a utilisation value for people with similar characteristics.

However, because of these characteristics, this classification may be valid for other populations on other continents, as the values found may correspond to an average for the world population.

The differences between the sexes should also be noted, as the values for males are individually lower than those for females. This means that, when indicating a surgical procedure for a male patient, the professional should pay attention to seeking the best result for the patient and not look for the value presented in the classification, which only has meaning when it comes to the patient's clinical complaint.

It frames an instrument to accompany the patient during their ageing process, just like the pictorial portraits created by Albrecht Durer, who began his self-portrait at the age of thirteen and did it until he could no longer paint[18] , recording his ageing.

Objectively, the classification proposed here will help plastic surgeons to formalise the follow-up of their patients and their results, whether surgical or not, as well as providing them with more data for differential diagnoses, such as in cases of palpebral pseudoptosis.

The objective measurement of the position of the tail of the eyebrow makes it possible to classify the degree of ptosis and advise on the need for surgical intervention, making it an important tool for diagnosing and proposing treatment in terms of harmonising the upper third of the face.

Bibliography

1- Bramly, Serge. Leonardo da Vinci. Rio de Janeiro, Imago, 1989.

2- Shaw RB Jr, Katzel EB, Koltz PF, Yaremchuk MJ, Girotto JA, Kahn DM, Langstein HN. Aging of the facial skeleton: aesthetic implications and rejuvenation strategies. Plast Reconstr Surg. 2011 Jan;127(1):374-83.

3- Matros E, Garcia JA, Yaremchuk MJ. Changes in eyebrow position and shape with aging. Plast Reconstr Surg. 2009 Oct;124(4):1296-301.

4- Gordon C. Aymar, The Art of Portrait Painting, Chilton Book Co., Philadelphia, 1967, p. 93.

5- Naif-de-Andrade NT, Hochman B, Naif-de-Andrade CZ, Ferreira LM. Computerised photogrammetry used to calculate the brow position index. Aesthetic Plast Surg. 2012 Oct;36(5):1047-51. doi: 10.1007/s00266-012-9961-7. Epub 2012 Aug 31.

6- Packiriswamy V, Kumar P, Bashour M. Photogrammetric analysis of eyebrow and upper eyelid dimensions in South Indians and Malaysian South Indians. Aesthet Surg J. 2013 Sep 1;33(7):975-82. doi:

10.1177/1090820X13503472. Epub 2013 Sep 9.

7- Jones BM, Lo SJ. The impact of endoscopic brow lift on eyebrow morphology, aesthetics, and longevity: objective and subjective measurements over a 5-year period. Plast Reconstr Surg. 2013 Aug;132(2):226e-238e. doi: 10.1097/PRS.0b013e3182958b9f.

8- Hamamoto AA, Liu TW, Wong BJ. Identifying ideal brow vector position: empirical analysis of three brow archetypes. Facial Plast Surg. 2013 Feb;29(1):76-82. doi: 10.1055/s-0033-1333841. Epub 2013 Feb 20.

9- Nahai FR. The varied options in brow lifting. Clin Plast Surg. 2013 Jan;40(1):101-4. doi: 10.1016/j.cps.2012.08.007. Epub 2012 Oct 23. Review.

10- Lee NG, Callahan AB, Migliori ME, Freitag SK. Minimally invasive approaches to eyebrow lifting. Int Ophthalmol Clin. 2013 Summer;53(3):47- 57. doi: 10.1097/IIO.0b013e31829053f6

11- Lee JW, Cho BC, Lee KY. Direct brow lift combined with suspension of the orbicularis oculi muscle. Arch Plast Surg. 2013 Sep;40(5):603-9. doi: 10.5999/aps.2013.40.5.603. Epub 2013 Sep 13.

12- Matai O, Lavezzo MM, Schellini SA, Padovani CR, Padovani CR. Evaluation of eyebrow position using angular measures]. Arq Bras Oftalmol. 2007 Jan-Feb;70(1):41-4. Portuguese.

13- Basic Notions and Concepts in Occlusion, Temporomandibular Dysfunction and Orofacial Pain; Helson José de Paiva and Collaborators; Livraria Santos Editora, 2008.

14- Atran, S. Cognitive foundations of natural history: towards an anthropology of science. Cambridge: Cambridge Univ. Press. 1990. xii+360 p. (ISBN 0-521-37293-3).

15- Hochman B, Nahas FX, Ferreira LM. [Photography in medical research]. Acta Cir Bras. 2005;20 Suppl 2:19-25. Epub 2005 Nov 4.

16- Hwang K. Surgical anatomy of the upper eyelid relating to upper blepharoplasty or blepharoptosis surgery. Anat Cell Biol. 2013 Jun;46(2):93- 100. doi: 10.5115/acb.2013.46.2.93. Epub 2013 Jun 30.

17- Fitzgerald R. Contemporary concepts in brow and eyelid aging. Clin Plast Surg. 2013 Jan;40(1):21-42. doi: 10.1016/j.cps.2012.08.005. Review.

18- John Hope-Hennessy, The Portrait in the Renaissance, Bollingen Foundation, New York, 1966, pp. 124-126.

CHAPTER 3

Surgical Correction for Ptosis of the Tail of the Eyelid

Frontotemporal minilifting to suspend the tail of the eyebrow: minimally invasive Reis-Sundfeld technique*

Dr Daniel Sundfeld Spiga Real

***Article published in the Brazilian Journal of Plastic Surgery**
- Rev. Bras. Cir. Plást. 2015;30(3):446-454

Facial ageing is multifactorial. Over time, the force of gravity, constant muscle contractions and loss of skin elasticity form lines in the frontal region, glabellar furrows and cause the brow to droop.[1,2]

The orbital region is an extremely expressive part of the face. The position of the eyebrow says a lot about facial expression. Depending on its shape and position, it gives off an air of tiredness, vigour or other moods. Ptosis of the eyebrow and eyelid is one of the main complaints during consultations[1,3] .

They usually occur after the age of 45 when the lateral region or tail of the supercilia shows a greater degree of ptosis, thus causing an accumulation of skin on the upper eyelids, sometimes surpassing the eyelashes[2,4] . Another common complaint, in addition to the aged appearance of the orbital region, is visual difficulty due to the reduction in the amplitude of the eyelid opening, causing a reduction in the visual field[3] .

Eyebrow ptosis results in the false appearance of excess upper eyelid skin. If it is not promptly recognised at the time of the physical assessment, it can lead to an inappropriate procedure for the patient, causing this ptosis to worsen by reducing the space between the eyebrow and the "ciliary level" through a conventional blepharoplasty[4] .

For this reason, a careful assessment must be carried out together with the morphological characteristics that contextualise the patient's complaints. Eyelid pseudoptosis caused by superciliary ptosis in patients who don't want more invasive surgeries and/or those that leave apparent marks on the eyebrows, inappropriately treated with blepharoplasty, will make passive eyelid closure difficult during sleep and can cause serious ocular impairment[3] .

There are numerous procedures and surgical techniques described for brow lift[5] . From 1919, when the first technique using elliptical excisions of the frontal and temporal regions was published, to the present day, procedures have undergone important advances, especially with the introduction of the endoscope .[5]

Among the techniques mentioned, Castanares' surgery stands out: through an elliptical excision of the skin just above the eyebrows (Castanares, 1964)[6] , or through small incisions on the sides of the eyebrows (mini Castanares), a lasting and desirable effect of raising the tail of the eyebrows is achieved[7] .

As a non-surgical alternative for repositioning the supercilium, it is possible to use botulinum toxin injections in the different depressor muscle groups and also lasers that redensify and contract the collagen, giving the ephemeral effect of elevating this region[8] .

Technique Description

The patients had their ptosis of the tail of the eyelid classified according to the definitions in Chapter 2 of this book and answered the body image index questionnaire[9] and were referred to the outpatient surgical setting.

Firstly, the markings are made according to the illustrations: Figures I and II in which the lines are delimited: mid-pupillary (MP), the line passing through the excantium parallel to the mid-pupillary (EC) and the line delimited by the excantium and the end of the eyebrow (ECFS).

Once these markings have been made, the digital examination marks out point X, which will be the vertex of the triangle and will determine how high the tail of the eyebrow will rise. This point is on a line parallel to the ECFS line that intersects the EC line with the highest part of the eyebrow.

Finally, the last vertex of the triangle is delimited by the intersection of a line parallel to the ECFS line and which crosses the intersection of the MP line with the highest portion of the eyebrow, as shown in Figures I and II.

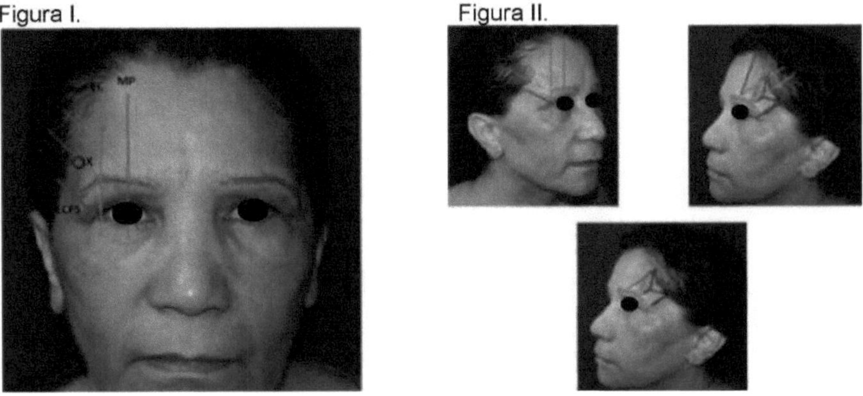

Figura I. Figura II.

Following the appointments, the patients were placed in the supine position, antiseptically treated with 2% chlorhexidine, given local anaesthetic solution (2% Xylocaine with vasoconstrictor) and sterile drapes were placed. First generation cephalosporins were used as antibiotic therapy.

After excision of the triangular contour of skin from the fronto-temporal region to the subdermal level, strict haemostasis was followed.

The next step was to use the technique proposed by these authors of making a subdermal stitch with colourless Mononylon 4.0 at the apex of the triangle towards the midpoint of the base. This allowed the tail of the eyebrow to be suspended up to the distance previously determined during clinical examination, using the measurement determined by the Frankfurt plane and the end of the tail of the eyebrow, as shown in Figure 1.

The others, according to the symmetry of the wound. Subsequently, the external stitches were made with Mononylon 5.0, separately. After this time, the effects were observed.

The above-mentioned procedures are repeated in the contralateral fronto-temporal region and at the end they are compared for symmetry. A micropore dressing is applied, preferably in skin colour. Patients should be followed up with regular visits.

At every return visit, patients should be photographed for later comparison, and the occurrence of complications such as infection, haematomas, epidermolysis, sensation of paresthesia, suture dehiscence, recurrence of superciliary ptosis and extrusion of threads should be assessed. Measurements should be taken directly, classifying the ptosis according to its degree from I to IV, between the Frankfurt Plane and the end of the tail of the eyebrow to control suspension effects, as shown in Graph I.

The measurement should be carried out according to the specifications in

Chapter 2 of this book, with the patients in an orthostatic position with a neutral gaze fixed on the horinzon and with the facial muscles relaxed. Use a digital caliper (precision 0.01mm; OTMT Machines, NY, USA) to measure the end point of the supercilium (FS) at the Frankfurt plane (PF) (Figure 1), drawing a line (X) that connects these points and makes a 90° angle with the Frankfurt plane (Figures 2a, 2b and 2c).

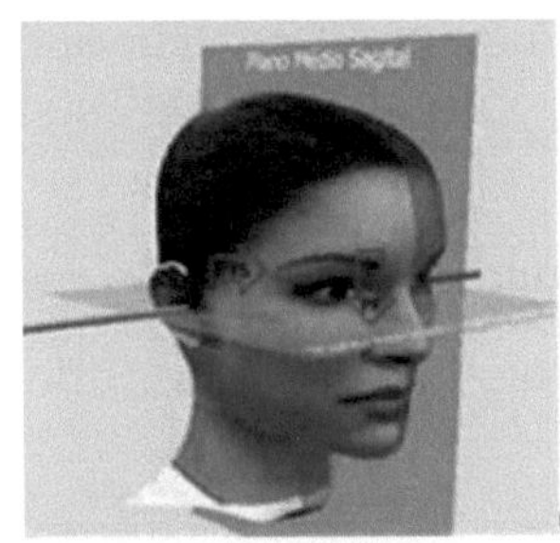

(Figura1).

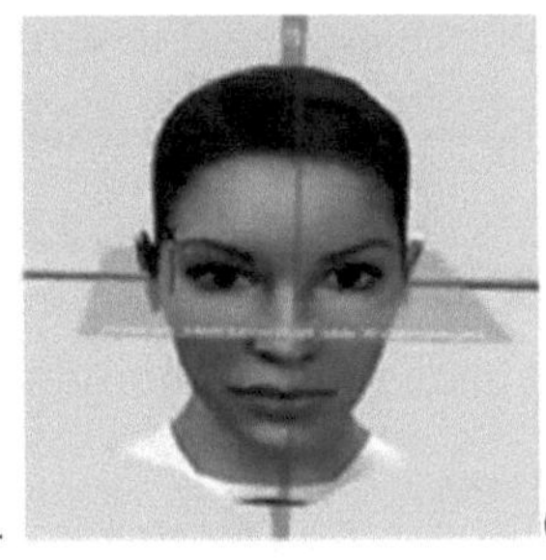

(Figura2a).

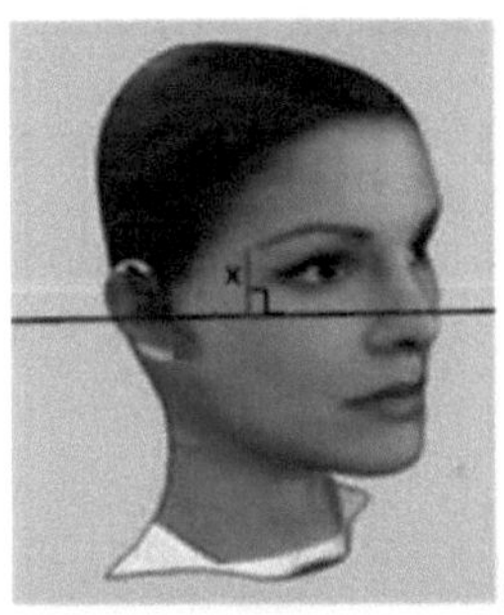

(Figura 2b).

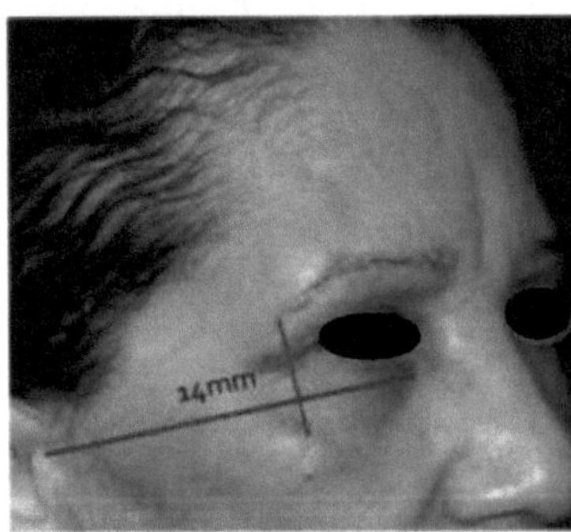

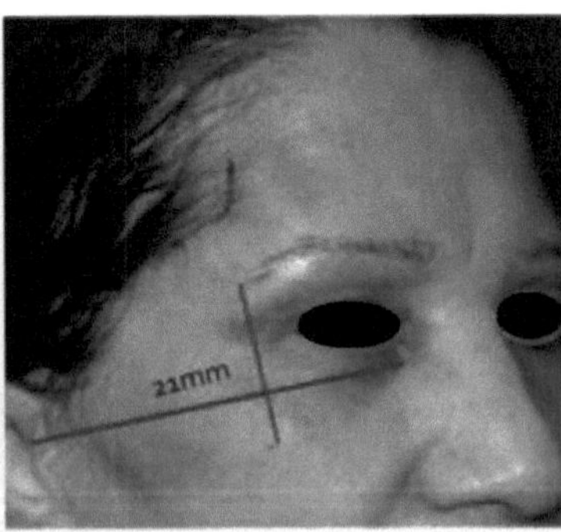

(Figura 2c).

As a definition, the Frankfurt Plane is the plane established by the lowest point of the orbital margin to the highest point of the external auditory canal[10] , which is why it is an important reference point, as it changes little with age, and is chosen as the fixed point for measurements.

The results and analyses of the questionnaires were plotted on graphs for better visibility.

In the initial measurements, the mean value was 13.3mm, with a median of 13mm among the ten patients. One month after surgery, the values identified were: mean 19.2mm and median 19mm. At the end of the sixth month, the values were: mean 18.9mm and median 18mm, while at the end of the 12th month of follow-up, the measurements were: mean 18.2mm and median 18mm. These results can be seen in Graph 1 below.

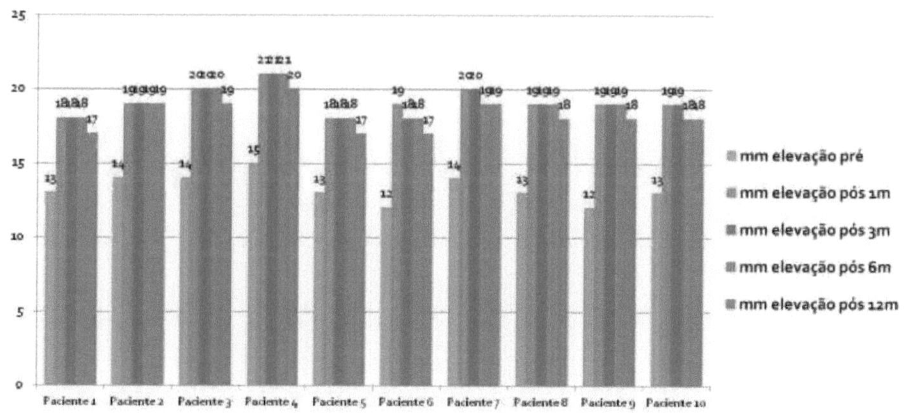

Graph 1. Degree of eyebrow tail elevation 12 months postoperatively.

With regard to the self-image satisfaction questionnaires, the results are shown below in graphs 2a and 2b, showing a significant improvement in patients' self-esteem, with 70% dissatisfied preoperatively and 90% extremely satisfied and satisfied six months after surgery.

pre Body Image Index

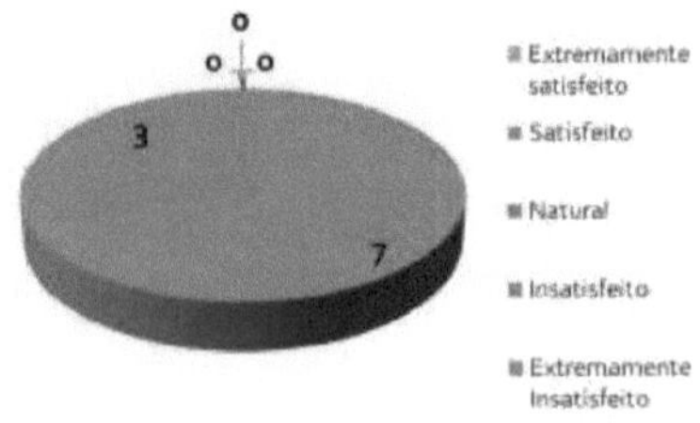

Graph 2a. Preoperative index.

Body Image Index after 6m

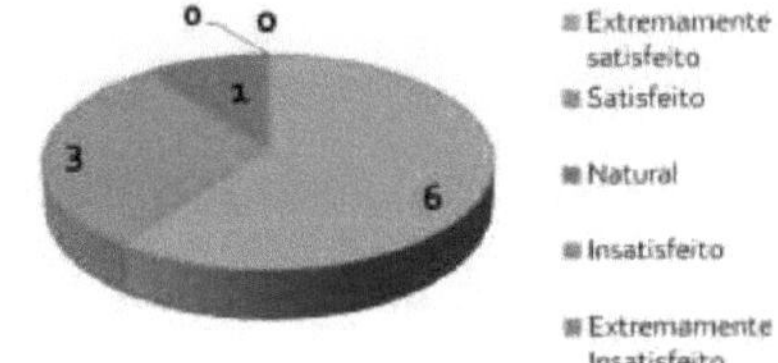

Graph 2b. 6-month post-operative index.

As a snapshot of surgical results, for a glimpse beyond the graphs, here is an example of a patient in pre-surgery and with a 12-month evolution (figure 3):

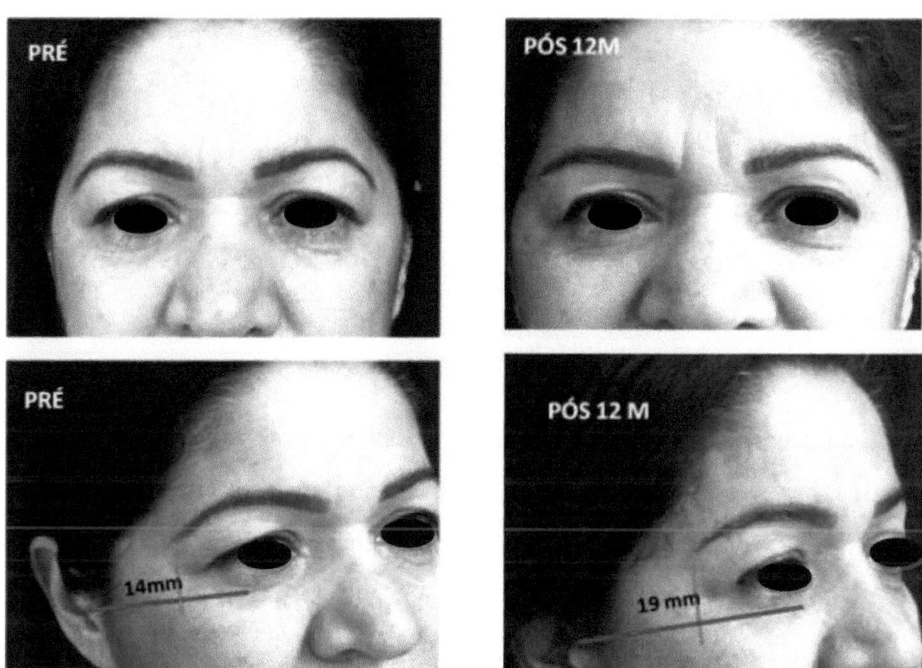

(Figure 3).

Literature Review

As an archetype, human beauty is represented mainly in the face, with all its nuances and expressions of feelings, as well as the appearance of the body's ageing stages. This demonstrates the great importance of facial expressions and the proportions of their constituents in men's social relationships and health.

In this context, the supercilium, especially its tail, represents, through its movements and placement, the sector with the greatest capacity to portray an individual's feelings as well as their ageing, as well characterised by the writer and artist Gordon C. Aymar: "the eyes are the place where the most complete, reliable and pertinent information about the person is seen.

subject. And the eyebrow can register, almost by itself, wonder, pity, fear, pain, cynicism, concentration, nostalgia, displeasure and hope, in infinite variations and combinations."[11] .

The Reis-Sundfeld fronto-temporal minilifting procedure aims to soften periocular wrinkles and reposition the eyebrow, restoring a more youthful appearance[12,13,14] . An important sign of ageing is the drooping of the eyebrow tail, which gives the face a sad look.

With the minimally invasive suspension described above, the eyebrow is lifted, as well as the adjacent upper eyelid tissue, resulting in a reduction in wrinkles, expression marks and sagging in the lateral region of the orbital and glabellar fissure.

Obtaining a satisfactory brow lift result requires a meticulous assessment of the position and characteristics of the tissues adjacent to the eyes, brow and frontal region[13,14] . The shape and bone structure of the face, the shape and height of the eyes in relation to the hair; the length and width of the upper 1/3, nose, mouth, eyelid, temples - all of these must be considered during the physical assessment of the face.[1,2,4]

The medial end of the eyebrow should start at the level of the ipsilateral nostril, and the space between them is equal to the distance between the eyes[1,4] . The lateral end of the eyebrow corresponds to an imaginary line from the nostril to the outer corner of the eye. The highest part of the curvature (arch) should be perpendicular to the outer side of the iris[1,2,4] .

These anatomical characteristics determine the need to adjust the elevation vector of the eyebrow tail for a more natural result. In the literature, some authors have carried out studies to try to determine the best elevation vector for the treatment of brow tail ptosis. These include the vectors recommended by Westmore,

Lamas and Anastasia, as presented in the article by Hamamoto et al[15] . In the technique proposed by this author, the vector used is similar to the one used by Anastasia which, in modern times, is characterised as the most accepted by specialists.

Patients who benefit from surgery using the technique proposed by the authors are those with sagging and ptosis in the region of the tail of the eyebrow, without eyelid excess, because if there is eyelid dermatochalasis, upper blepharoplasty surgery should also be performed.

This technique uses the mid-pupillary line, the lateral edge of the orbital fissure and the lateral end of the eyebrow as markers and parameters. A triangular incision is made in the fronto-temporal region with the base of the triangle at the hair insertion, with the aim of camouflaging the suture line. There are no specific absolute contraindications for this surgery.

The choice of this technique, rather than a possible rhytidoplasty or video-assisted frontal surgery, which are more extensive surgeries, should be made according to the surgical indication, bearing in mind the advantages and limitations that this procedure offers.

There are techniques in the literature that aim to rejuvenate the face, especially the eye area. However, compared to the technique described here, they are more complex to perform, using non-absorbable threads to fix the flaps after extensive flap dissection[13,14] . Fronto-temporal minilifting allows for a suspension of the tail of the eyebrow comparable to the Castanares and video-assisted frontal lift techniques, when assessing the level of suspension of the tail of the eyebrow, but without the stigma of a supraciliary scar compared to Castanares and with a smaller size compared to the video-assisted frontal lift.

Another factor that stands out is the fact that the results can be seen immediately after the procedure and can last for more than 12 months.

Also as an adjuvant to the surgical procedure, botulinum toxin can be used in the frontal region depressors with synergistic action in the rejuvenation of the upper third of the face resulting from frontotemporal minilifting[13] for an optimised effect of the results obtained. This application should be carried out two weeks before the procedure to reduce tension in the scar in the immediate post-operative period and until type III collagen is converted into type I, promoting greater scar resistance.

Conclusion

Considering the above, it should be noted that the proposed technique is an excellent option for the treatment of ptosis of the eyebrow tail because it is a minimally invasive, low-cost procedure, with no need for nosocomial infrastructure and minimal or no complications.

It is easy to mark, with well-determined points, making it reproducible for surgeons. The results showed an average elevation comparable to the current standard techniques, video-assisted and coronal frontoplasty, with results lasting 12 months.

From the above, we propose a simple, reproducible surgical technique, with local blockage, and above all, with a satisfactory repair result for the positioning of the tail of the eyebrow, when properly indicated, re-establishing the harmony of the face, especially its upper third, and bringing light and vitality to the gaze.

We stress that, as in all the other chapters, there is no ideal technique. Each case must be considered unique, with diagnoses carried out in a ubiquitous manner and the proposal of the treatment that is best suited to the patient's complaints and diagnosed problems, with a view to facial harmonisation that is both beautiful and functional.

Never forget that plastic surgery is a medical speciality, and that it is a means to an end! Plastic Surgery doesn't promise results, but it does have the necessary tools to treat changes in the shape and functionality of parts.

Bibliography

1) Naif-de-Andrade NT, Hochman B, Naif-de-Andrade CZ, Ferreira LM. Computerised photogrammetry used to calculate the brow position index. Aesthetic Plast Surg. 2012 Oct;36(5):1047-51.
2) Feser DF, Grundl M, Eisenmann-Klein M, Prantl L. Attractiveness of eyebrow position and shape in females depends on the age of the beholder. Aesth Plast Surg.2007;31:154-60.
3) Knize DM. Anatomic concepts for brow lift procedures. Plast Reconstr Surg. 2009Dec;124(6):2118-26. doi: 10.1097/PRS.0b013e3181bd0726.
4) Griffin GR, Kim JC. Ideal female brow aesthetics. Clin Plast Surg. 2013 Jan;40(1):147-55. doi: 10.1016/j.cps.2012.07.003. Epub 2012 Sep 8.

5) Paul MD. The evolution of the brow lift in aesthetic plastic surgery. Plast Reconstr Surg. 2001 Oct;108(5):1409-24.
6) Castanares S. Forehead wrinkles, glabellar frown and ptosis of the eyebrows. Plast Reconstr Surg. 1964;34:406-13.
7) Vinas JC, Caviglia C, Cortinas JL. Forehead rhytidoplasty and brow lifting. Plast Reconstr Surg. 1976;57:445-54.
8) Punthakee X, Keller GS, Vose JG, Stout W. New technologies in aesthetic blepharoplasty and brow-lift surgery. Facial Plast Surg. 2010 Aug;26(3):260-5. doi: 10.1055/s-0030-1254337. Epub 2010 Jun 3.
9) Melega, MP. Psychological Aspects of the Plastic Surgery Patient. Plastic Surgery - Fundamentals and Art. Ed Kooga; Vol I, pg 221-7, 2002.
10) Basic Notions and Concepts in Occlusion, Temporomandibular Dysfunction and Orofacial Pain; Helson José de Paiva and Collaborators; Livraria Santos Editora, 2008.
11) Gordon C. Aymar, The Art of Portrait Painting, Chilton Book Co., Philadelphia, 1967, p. 93.
12) Arneja JS, Larson DL, Gosain AK. Aesthetic and reconstructive brow lift: current techniques, indications, and applications. Ophthal Plast Reconstr Surg. 2005 Nov;21 (6):405-11.
13) Centurión P, Romero C. Lateral brow lift: a surgical proposal. Aesthetic Plast Surg. 2010 Dec;34(6):745-57. doi: 10.1007/s00266-010- 9537-3. Epub 2010 Jun 30.
14) Alex JC. Aesthetic considerations in the elevation of the eyebrow. Facial Plast Surg. 2004 Aug;20(3):193-8.
15) Hamamoto AA, Liu TW, Wong BJ. Identifying ideal brow vector

position: empirical analysis of three brow archetypes. Facial Plast Surg. 2013 Feb;29(1):76-82. doi: 10.1055/s-0033-1333841. Epub 2013 Feb 20.

Completion of the work

In framing the outcome of this work, it is clear that at no point did we intend to exhaust the marvellous and challenging world of facial plastic surgery, as it is imponderable.

Plastic surgery, like other medical specialities, is constantly evolving, and here we quote the eminent pre-Socratic philosopher Heraclitus of Ephesus, who defines in his thoughts that "everything flows", the world in perpetual motion. Such is the art of body sculpture, which seeks to bring to the surface the beauty that lies at the heart of each one of us, as well as having the strenuous duty of making functional what once was no longer functional.

In this kaleidoscopic progression, plastic surgery, at every historical moment, acts in an incessant search for the harmony of the parts to build a whole in golden proportion!

The aim of this book is to bring a small drop of water from an immensity of knowledge from the oceans of science, to arouse curiosity about knowledge and the production of knowledge.

We hope to achieve our goal of making researchers of all our readers, as well as spreading our contributions to science, especially to Plastic Surgery and all the patients who will benefit from them.

We'd like to say "see you soon" to our readers, and we hope to meet you in new chapters of this fundamental work of art: Plastic Surgery!

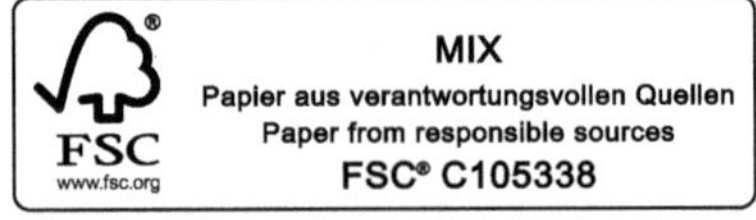

Printed by Books on Demand GmbH, Norderstedt / Germany